Life After 70
Upsides and Positives
By Lillie Gincard

ISBN: 1475148879

Published by: www.Createspace.com

Printed in the United States of America

For Mom

Contents

Preface

I met Rose Bickman through a friend of mine who runs a very successful bed and breakfast place called *The Hideaway,* in Connecticut. Rose is a 76-year-old retired bank employee. She's been living in a senior hi-rise building in New York City since her husband of 46 years passed away. Rose does not agree with what she calls the *rocking-chair* mentality and lifestyle that some of society slots people into once they pass the age of 55.

When my husband passed away two years ago, I retired from my editing position and now spend most of my time writing about the people I meet in my travels. I go to *The Hideaway* once a year to relax and gather new material for whatever I happen to be working on at the time.

I've met quite a few retirees who have different views on aging and dealing with the many situations we face in this changing world. Rose's attitude impressed me so much that I decided to give her ideas a voice, as well as those of some of her friends, and many of the women I interviewed briefly at random.

So, here you'll have a few pearls, and some personal comments relating to aging, as well as a few laughs, in this collection of *Upsides and positives* to life after 70.

I must say that at 74 years old, I hadn't really taken the time to analyze the aging process in such a completely positive way, but as Rose said to me, "You've just been too busy *worrying* about growing old that you forgot to take the time to enjoy it."

There are downsides to *any* life for sure, Rose says. Like living alone and having no one to laugh with when you're watching *Shrek, Toy Story, Finding Nemo, or Shark Tale.* And getting older is never easy, because with the aging comes aches and pains, both physical and mental. Loved ones and friends die and leave you behind to face life alone; Some of society ostracizes you in many ways by lumping you in the *elderly/rocking-chair* slot, and worst of all, something called CRS (<u>C</u>an't <u>R</u>emember <u>S</u>hit) begins to take over your life.

Rose and her friends, and the women I talked to, say there are enough negatives to aging to fill up your days and nights, if you concentrate on them. But when you weigh all the *downsides and negatives* to life after 70 against the *upsides and positives*, you can find that you actually have the advantage in many ways. And you'll find that there are so many more upsides and positives, you'll forget about the negatives and downsides.

Besides, as Rose says, there are always enough other people to fill the seats on the negative train. And the expression "Every cloud has a silver lining" is exactly what your senior years are. No matter how dark the lonely hours get sometime, no matter how big the black cloud of hopelessness, despair, or depression that sweeps over you once in a while, or how often CRS creeps into your days, Rose says there are bright spots to be found.

You just have to open your heart and mind and make the effort to look for them.

Acknowledgements

Heartfelt thanks to my two Jewels Skye and CC, two of the wisest people I've ever known, for all that they add to my life, and to *their* Jewels and their Jewels' Jewels.

PART ONE

Counting Your Blessings

1.   Waking Up in the Morning

You get to make the day your own special miracle. You get to choose without asking anyone else's opinion:

a) Oh, woe is me. Another day.

b) Yippee! Another day!

It may not always be easy to choose, especially if you're grieving the loss of a loved one or a friend. But there's always that *Yippee!* choice: ***You woke up this morning!!***

2.   You're not waiting in line at the Crematorium or the burial site

3.   God and your family love you even though you may be a pain in the butt sometimes

4.   Medicare covers most of your medical bills, and you have prescription coverage for co-pay

5.   No More Birth Control Pills!

But even if you did get *with child,* you could take the spotlight away from the 67-year-old Romanian woman, who in January, 2005 became the oldest woman ever known to give birth.

And companies would flock to your door to offer everything from formula to college scholarships, in exchange for an interview and a chance to advertise their products.

Then when there's a break in the crazy publicity, you can

9

check yourself into a mental hospital for observation!

6. Senior Discounts

Many businesses offer senior discounts on: car rentals, travel costs, hotel fees, and many, many more services and products.

And your local businesses like *Dunkin' Donuts* may offer them, as well as some bus companies. Be proud when you ask, "Do you give senior discounts?"

7. Free stuff

It can be a struggle living on a fixed budget, but riding public transportation free can open up opportunities for entertainment, and adventure.

For example, in Rhode Island if your annual income is below a certain level, public transportation is *free*. And there's no need to ever try to cheat if your income happens to increase above the minimum level, because even then you can still benefit by only paying half fare.

It makes a huge difference if you like exploring new places, or visiting the malls and getting a really good work-out walking around. In Rhode Island you can spend a whole day touring around the state with connecting buses at the Kennedy Plaza bus depot, without putting a big dent in your budget.

8. Senior Housing

If you don't happen to own your own home, this benefit is a God-send. In these government-subsidized buildings your rent is calculated based on your annual income and expenses, and you get to live in a secure, immaculate place you can call home; you can just *live*.

And, you rest easy knowing that if you live long enough to get excessively feeble and can't even remember what the hell CRS is, there's still hope: *Assisted Living*! You can still maintain some sense of independent living, with help. At these facilities you have your meals prepared, you get help with everyday things like laundry, house cleaning, shopping, and much more.

Extra perks in your senior hi-rise building:

--A full-service clinic on the first floor of your hi-rise building, with a doctor, and a sympathetic nurse who makes you feel welcome, and talks calmly to you even when you whine about this and that as it relates to getting old and taking medications

--A well-kept laundry room on every floor

--Immaculate building hallways, and common areas

--A Meals On Wheels site in a spacious, comfortable dining-room

--24-hour security guards

--A fully-equipped small gym that's open to tenants at all times

9.   Not having to watch the clock every minute. The fact that you're *still here* is all that matters, no matter what time it is

10.   No more *multi-tasking*. There's time enough to just take one step at a time, complete one task at a time, enjoy one meal at a time, etc.

11.   Retirement

After working most of your life, going to bed with a clearly-planned day ahead of you for five days a week is suddenly gone. For some people, after raising children and possibly losing a mate early in life, it can be very difficult. Suddenly, you slot yourself into the cubby hole most of society has carved out for retirees like you: the rocking chair, waiting for the invitation from St. Peter.

After a few months of annoying the hell out of everyone and lamenting about your situation, you can emerge from the cocoon of self-pity and depression.

You can sign up with a temp agency for part-time work. Ugh! Didn't you retire so that you could have time to do all the things you never had time for when you were working five days a week (and week-ends for some of us). Well, now all you have to do is make plans and take advantage of the activities available especially for you.

First, when that madness about the part-time job wears off, you can cut up a bunch of little slips of paper and write different activities on them; include your favorite activities and hobbies.

Put the slips of paper in a jar (your *choice jar*). Be sure to add slips that say *couch day,* and *folderol.*

Each morning choose an activity from the jar.

When you go to bed at night you'll know there'll be a surprise waiting for you because you won't remember what activities you've written on the little slips of paper anyway. Immediately after you wrote out the slips and put them in the jar CRS took over, so you'll be surprised every time you take a slip from the choice jar.

After a while you'll be so busy with things you never had the time to do while you were working, you'll wind up going days without choosing an activity from the jar. You'll soon become a pro at the retiree business and your days will be filled with things like helping out your neighbors, volunteering, spending time with other retired friends, or with family, going to the discounted movie, reading for hours at a time uninterrupted, having more spontaneous sex with your partner, etc.

But once in a while you can still choose an activity from the jar just for old time's sake. And if those old feelings of *woe-is-me* start to creep up again, watch a full hour of The Jerry Springer show and you'll thank God for YOU!!! How does that sound?

Of course, if you're a natural social butterfly you already have your activities planned out. And, there are so many groups and organizations that offer activities for seniors if you're willing to put forth the effort to search them out. And most senior independent and assisted living facilities offer a range of activities for you, carefully planned by a person hired specifically for this purpose.

12.   **Hobbies**

Indulging in hobbies never fails to chase away Arthritis and Pity Party guests, and, if you're *crafty,* you can sell your items on-line, or at flea markets, or donate them to church bazaars, or groups like *Teen Challenge,* or *Big Sisters, etc.*

Besides, having a hobby that fills up a bunch of your leisure time will save you money because you won't have time to watch all those infomercials, and buy the gadgets they advertise because they look so *handy.*

13.   You recognize the old person in your mirror

14.   Not having to go out in the cold, or heat to punch a clock

15.   Bouncing back five times when life's circumstances knock you down four times

16.   Having enough supplies in the fridge and cupboard to last you until your next social security or pension check comes in another week

17.   Drawing on your deep-seeded inner strength that lets you find your way back through the maze of negativity and obstacles that occasionally block your path

18.   The knife of envy eludes you among your friends

19.   Surviving six whole months without having to be poked, prodded, x-rayed, or stuck to have multiple tubes of blood drawn

20.   Friends who are older than you; you get to pick their brains for their secrets to aging well

21.   A doctor who actually listens to you and lets you explain how you feel *before* he takes out the prescription pad

22.   Remembering precisely where you left your reading glasses

23.   Not having to worry about having anything *lifted, sucked, implanted, puffed up, or dyed.* You can let your body age naturally if you prefer, by eating healthy, staying active, and choosing to savor all the joys in life possible

24.   A partner who cleans the specks off the bathroom mirror after flossing

25.   Checking the pockets of a jacket before adding it to the washing machine and discovering a $20 bill you had forgotten about

26.   A partner who actually respects you, despite the fact that you're seven years older than they are

27.   Bus drivers who lower the bus for you without you having to ask, so that your knees don't cry when you get on or off the bus

28.   Embracing the advice of *Wilma Melville* - - A rescue dog trainer - - who says that if you're breathing, it's not too late; get up and get going, she says; age is just a number

29.   <u>**Libman© Mops**</u>

You don't have to bend over too much and put your hands in the water to wring them out

30.   <u>**The ability to forgive**</u>

One evening you're out at an elegant restaurant with your new partner of five years (after recovering from a divorce from a physically-abusive husband). During dessert you spot the ex-husband waiting on tables and looking depressed and down-trodden. There's no trace of the egotistical, self-serving, abusive man who used to put you down at every opportunity.

As you're returning to your table after a trip to the ladies' room, the ex-husband steps in front of you and says quietly, "How are you, Gloria? You look wonderful." "I'm fine, Dan," you answer as you resist the urge to whack him across the face with your purse. "I was a fool to treat you the way I did," he says, and he actually seems on the verge of tears.

You notice that his eyes are blood-shot, his once-handsome body is lumpy, and he is slouching forward like a very old man, but he's only 73. Your heart goes out to him as he says, "You were the best thing that I had and I mistreated you. I'm truly sorry for that. If that's your new husband, I hope he knows what a lucky man he is."

As he starts to walk away, you take his arm and make eye contact. "I forgive you, Dan," you say, "and I wish you happiness." You hug him and whisper, "God bless you." As you walk away you feel the burden of carrying around all the hate and resentment you felt towards him slip away, and you send up a silent prayer for him.

31.   A partner who supports your idea of separate bedrooms. They have their *own* private space, and you have yours. In your space you can wallow in your little idiosyncrasies, like lining your dresser top with miniature collectible cat figures, and your partner can choose to leave their socks and underwear in a pile on the floor whenever they choose. This arrangement can save a relationship if one of you snores, or one of you is what people call a *T and T* (a toss and turner).

And even though most nights one of you slips in with the other one, there are those rare occasions when you both appreciate the option of having your separate sleeping space.

32.   Unexpected dinner invitations from friends when the pity party guests are clamming at your door

33.   A friend who comforts you with a warm hug and encouraging words, without any ulterior motives

34.   Most days you know exactly who you are, where you are, what day or year it is, who the president is, etc.

35.   On your 71st birthday you receive:

--19 phone calls and text messages from family and friends with happy birthday wishes

--A beautiful bouquet of flowers from your daughter

--A visit from your son and three of his children who bring Chinese food and a birthday cake.

PART TWO

Grown-up children/grand children/Great-grandchildren

A. Grown-up Children

1.   When we're raising our children, we fight off demons, make sacrifices, and try to teach them right from wrong, and a multitude of "how to's". We become martyrs in our struggles raising them. Our love is like lead; it cannot be chipped, shattered, or broken no matter how many times it's hit with life's struggles, challenges, disappointments, etc. We don't expect gratitude or reciprocation for doing what is required of us while we're raising them.

But what do they do the minute they learn to walk by themselves? They begin walking away from us in so many ways. First they learn to feed and clothe themselves without our help; they learn to cross the street by themselves without us holding their hands and telling them constantly to look both ways; they start going to school and manage to last a whole seven hours without our guidance. Soon after that they go to that holy institution called high school, where they discover *crushes*, and they no longer want you to kiss or hug them in public; in fact they would prefer it if they weren't seen in public with you at all!

Oh, it gets worse. Then they have the colossal nerve to grow into their adult life without you controlling every aspect of their lives and guiding them through the hoops. They become successful and actually live a life of their own in an apartment or house some distance away from you (sometimes in a totally different state!) And get this, they pay the rent or mortgage without your help.

THEN, they have families of their own, bring the children to see you often, and one day you hear them telling their children some of the same things you used to tell *them* when you were trying to guide them in the right direction. You see them hugging their children and showing them how to love, and be a worthwhile and caring human being, and *you forgive them for growing up!!*

Because finally you realize that you've been angry at them for actually doing what you prayed for them to do: *grow up and become independent.* And you also realize that no matter how independent they've become now, they will *always need you*, just in different ways, and that fact in itself is so comforting because:

--You become like a couch cushion that supports their back when they sit down

--They will need you to cook their favorite meal or dessert just the way you used to when they were little

--They will need you to just listen when they want to vent, because they know they can trust you with their deepest feelings, and concerns

--They'll need those special *Mommy* hugs, or *Dad* embraces once in a while

And there will be so many other ways in which they will *always* need you that will crop up often, as long as you live.

2. It's raining cats and dogs out. You're fighting an awful cold, and the pity party guests are clamming to get started. You keep them at bay by reading Agatha Christie's *Endless Night* again about the young man who didn't know when he was really in love.

By chapter four you start to reminisce about when your children were small enough to need you, so you haul out the family photos and start flipping through a few albums. When you run across a few pictures of the time you took them on a trip to Washington, you invite the pity party guests in.

Five minutes after you relinquish your self control to the pity party guests your cell phone signals a text message coming through from your daughter who lives in New Jersey (you live in Rhode

Island). The short message gives your heart a squeeze as you read it: *"Yes, mommy, I think about you every day xoo."*

In two seconds the pity party guests are chased out and you start working on your Christmas list, even though it's only April 3rd.

3. Fighting the blues and waiting for Hurricane Irene to knock down the trees outside your apartment building some time within the next 24 hours, you get a text message from your son who invites you out to dinner at a Chinese buffet with him and his son.

4. A son who takes you to dinner at a fancy restaurant on your 79th birthday, and has a real conversation with you. When an acquaintance of his stops at your table to say hello and asks your son who you are he says, "This is my best girl."

5. A daughter and son-in-law who take you to Disneyland for 4 days, all expenses paid.

6. Sometimes we may feel that our grown children forget that we still need to feel *needed*, even though we no longer have to work two jobs trying to keep body and soul together while trying to carve out time to spend with them.

But if we start to feel neglected, we'll remind ourselves that they now have their own families to work two jobs for in order to survive in this collapsing economy, and still they find the time for these perks, specifically for us:

--They give us money

--They take us out to lunch and to dinner

--They come over on Christmas day with gifts, lots of gifts

--They send us text messages with a smiley face and lots of x's and o's to tell us they love us, and always on the days we feel the loneliest, or the most un-needed

--They call us up out of the blue and say "Just checking on you."

--They never forget our birthday

--They send us gifts just for G.P. (general principles)

--*They give us money*

7.   <u>Nostalgia</u>

--Stumbling across a Valentine's Day card from your son that he made in school in the first grade

--Finding the first letter your 40-year-old daughter wrote you when she first discovered pencil and paper go together. It had lots of scraggly lines that she said reads "I love you, Mommy."

8.   <u>Conquering the Empty-Nest Syndrome</u>

You're a widow. Your grown daughter gets married and moves to another state. Six months later your son moves out of the house. Empty nest syndrome sets in and takes over your life and you begin searching for information about adopting, in a desperate search for someone who needs you.

A friend sets you up with her handsome, gentlemanly neighbor and you engage in a whirlwind spring romance. Dinners at romantic bistros, movie dates to see romantic movies like *Why Did I Get Married?,* walks in the park, etc., etc.

Another friend invites you to dinner. Their three children ages 17 to 27 still live at home and she tells you she's envious of you because, "… you're free, your children have left home and you have your life to yourself now." You lament that that is not the case, and you want to adopt. "What the hell is wrong with you?" she says.

The next day Federal Express delivers an important letter from your new man. You delay opening it for hours because you've heard horror stories about text-message break- ups, and you think maybe this letter contains a break-up message.

Finally, you get a glass of wine and sit down to open the letter. Inside is a paid Amtrak ticket to New York with the message: "Had to travel suddenly for business; will you join me for the weekend?" Woo Hoo. No kids to arrange baby-sitting for, no responsibilities, no worries except what to wear and whether or not there's time to get your hair done.

B. Grandchildren, and Great Grandchildren

1. One of life's gratifying experiences after having your own children, is the lofty position of *Granny*. We're held in high esteem by our grandchildren and great-grandchildren and we sometimes, almost, maybe, just a little bit maybe, feel guilty. But then we sit back and enjoy our placement on the *Granny Throne*.

It can also be heart-breaking to watch your children suffer the same *naughtiness,* from *their* children that they put us through.

And how can anything compete with the mere fact that you actually lived long enough to see your own children become grandparents? Of course, that makes you a great-granny and you get to brag about your miracles, and annoy anyone close enough with pictures and stories about their brilliance.

During those brief moments when we're off our *Granny* throne of honor, opportunities for pity parties abound.

Case in point: It's a cold, rainy day and you haven't spoken to anyone for five days; you're a widow, living alone. No chance of going out in the rain for a walk. Gloom hovers, and you can't stave off the pity party that lasts three hours, with you crying about being used up, no one needing you anymore, you're alone, no one loves you, no one cares, yada, yada, yada. Every negative thought possible comes to your pity party.

Upside: Just when all hope seems lost, you get a call from your daughter's oldest son (he's 25) asking you what you're doing.

"I'm cooking," you say. (You can't tell him you're having a pity party that might last all day.)

While you're chatting on the cell phone with him there's a knock at your door. When you open the door, it's the grandson you're talking to, on his cell phone. He's standing there with a bag of take-out from *Dave & Buster's*, and behind him are three of your son's children. Ha Ha.

You eat, talk, they play games on PS2 while you sit on your throne and Granny-up the situation. You're totally exhausted when they leave and you're the happiest Granny in the universe. It takes you an hour to clean up, but *Pity party be damned!!!*

2.   <u>Particularly Gratifying Granny Moments</u>

a) Your 12-year-old granddaughter tells you you're cool

b) Watching the *Shrek* series with your grandchildren

c) A grandson brings a friend over for some of your famous chocolate chip cookies

d) Babysitting the grandchildren for a week-end; then *sending them home*

OR

After nine hours of food, games, fun, and reminiscing, *the grandchildren are picked up.*

e) Realizing that our grandchildren and/or great-grandchildren are *other people's children*

f) A letter from a 6-year grandson saying you're the best Granny in the world

g) A ribbon from a grandson that says "World's Greatest Grandma"

h) Your 16-year-old artistic granddaughter takes a piece of fabric-coated art wire and shapes it into a heart and gives it to you

i) Your 19-year-old grandson gives you a kiss when he's leaving after a visit. You used to have to pay him a dollar to get a kiss, when he was seven

j) A granddaughter who calls you up occasionally "…just to say hello."

k) A plaque from a granddaughter that reads in part "…then God set the bar really high and created grandmas…"

l) A granddaughter who graduates from medical school third in her class. She's valedictorian at the ceremony and in her speech she credits her mother and you for her achievements

m) The first time your 5-year-old great-grandson says "…Great-Great Granny, I love you."

n) Remembering that Grannies have magical powers and we can dispense love droplets in the form of praise and encouragement, and offer our Queenly shoulders to cry on. Often we can make a tiny heart swell with feelings of special *Granny Love.*

And when we dispense advice, we remember to temporarily step down from the Granny Throne to the lowly position of an outsider, because after all: *They are other people's children*, even though we are ultimately responsible for their very existence.

We remember our chief assignment while on our Granny Throne is to dispense love, and encouragement to "Eat your vegetables, and be good to mom and dad."

We've raised our little angels. Now all we have to do is occupy our Granny throne and wait for the blessed opportunity to once again give advice or a shoulder to cry on, to our *own* grown-up angels again when they need us.

o) Your 36-year-old grandson who's a doctor drops by unexpectedly and takes you out to dinner. During dinner he asks about you and how you're getting along since your husband passed away (only a few months ago). And he listens with genuine concern and interest.

When he takes you home, he takes out the garbage, rinses up the few dishes in the sink, and straightens up a few things in the living room. By the time he leaves you feel so loved and cared for you don't even notice the creaking sounds Arthritis is making in your knees by the time you go to bed.

PART THREE

A. Age Defiance

1.   You go out one morning around 6:00 a.m. for your regular walk and some young punk tries to snatch your little purse you carry around your waist. There's no one around, the streets are empty except for a few cars whizzing by, so the punk thinks you're at his mercy.

Upside: The punk doesn't know that your oldest grandson taught you a few karate moves when he was only 7 years old. So you give the punk a swift kick in the family jewels, then when he bends over you whack him across the neck and put your foot on his back when he falls down. While he's trying to cradle his family jewels and massage his neck at the same time, you call 911 on your cell phone and report the thwarted robbery. Meanwhile, a concerned motorist stops and offers her help. She waits with you for the police to arrive.

When the police arrive and see all 125 pounds of your 5, 2 frame subduing the burly almost-crook, they invite you to a senior's meeting to help teach other seniors how to protect themselves from would-be muggers.

Wait, there's more. While at the meeting, you meet a very handsome, successful, single senior who asks for your phone number. Ha Ha. He He.

2.   Mango facials - - You rub the fresh mango seed over your face and let it dry for about 20 minutes, then carefully wipe it off with a very warm washcloth. Best pure facial ever, and it makes your skin tingle.

3.   Olive oil facial cleanser/make-up remover -- Rub a generous amount of olive oil on your face, then remove it with a very warm washcloth.

4.   Super foods: Salmon, mangos, pinto beans, sweet potatoes, raw almonds, kale, dried cherries

5.   Bringing your own cultivated brand of sunshine to a party

6.   Singing out loud without caring what you sound like

7.   Smiling at a total stranger without worrying about what they think's wrong with you

8.   Thong underwear from your partner, who has seen you naked

9.   If you're single: Recurring dreams about a Mustang Ranch for women where you can choose a Denzel Washington or a Harrison Ford clone

10.   <u>New Adventures</u>

Adventuring out of your comfort zone two weeks after your 78th birthday you dress up and walk into a bar alone - - for the first time in your life - - and order a drink at the bar. You sit there at the bar with your Kindle, reading and sipping your Hennessy. Three men try to pick you up and you discourage them all with the very useful: "I'm waiting for someone."
After your second Hennessy and a few interesting chats with the bartender during his free moments, you say, "I guess I've been stood up." You tip the bartender generously, saunter out of the bar, drive home and write about your adventure in your journal, hoping that when they finally open the Mustang Ranch for women, the men in the bar who tried to pick you up will work there.
(P.S. This won't work if you're in a committed relationship.)

11.   The slip of paper from your *choice jar* that says *FOLDEROL,* which means you're free to indulge in nonsensical things without the slightest concern about what other people think. You can play with your games and dolls all day if you want to, or you can play computer games until you pass out.

(P.S. - - To avoid getting calluses on your butt, take frequent 10-minute exercise breaks every so often: Walk up and down the hall if it's raining out; work out with weights; do stretches, touching your toes and that sort of thing.)

12.   You tube

      - High frequency music
      - Cats Playing Patty-Cake, and voices that tell you what they were saying

13.   This morning your partner said, "You were fabulous last night."

14.   Being able to sleep in the nude without the slightest concern about where things on your body are defying gravity

15.   You're retired, living alone. Your first volunteer appointment isn't until late afternoon. You roll over and retrieve the emergency supply of Oreos in the nightstand drawer.
      After six cookies you paddle bare feet and nude to the kitchen for a glass of cold milk. Then you brush away the morning breath, now somewhat subdued by the cookies, and start behaving like the adult you are.

16.   A visit to the zoo in your volunteer role as a surrogate Granny, with two seven-year-olds. You eat hot dogs and ice-cream and hear fantastic knock-knock jokes, and tell a few of your own that you've been saving up

17.   When you're alone, enjoying your second childhood, playing with your dolls, coloring in your special coloring book that you keep hidden in a drawer

18.   Keeping the *little grey cells* active with puzzles and brain-teasing games

19.   <u>**Your private feel-good TV. shows:**</u>

>   *-Sesame Street*
>   *-Word Girl*
>   *-Curious George*
>   *-The Cat In The Hat Knows A Lot About That*
>   *-Martha Speaks*

20.   Only one person who you trust with your life knows that Elmo is one of the loves of your life, with The Cookie Monster running a very close second.

21.   Louise Solomon yoga DVD's

22.   You agree to let your partner take tastefully naughty pictures of you (You're 76; he's 78). A week later your devious partner posts them on facebook. *Mortification* barely begins to describe your embarrassment.

>   <u>**Upside (Heck, yeah there's one)**</u>

You get a message via facebook from an agent who wants to take you on as a client. He knows of a magazine editor looking for "…fabulous-looking seniors…", to do a photo shoot for their magazine.
        So after you kick the skunk partner to the curb you go to lunch with your new agent, and begin a new and exciting career, or part-time job: your choice!

23.   At 76 you can still do the funky chicken, and the twist

24.   A live show with The Chippendale Dancers

25.   <u>**Exercise**</u> - At 77 you can still walk two miles a day, climb stairs, touch your toes without bending your knees, and do 15 squats without passing out.

26.   Whistles and *wolf* noises from workers when you're walking pass a construction site

27.   Younger hot guys trying to hit on you.

B. Beating Arthritis

1.   You have a particularly troublesome day, starting with that hateful monster, Arthritis. When you wake up you have to hobble to the shower and let the hot water warm up your bones enough so you can go about your day. You take your blood pressure medication, then later eat your healthy breakfast of oatmeal topped with blueberries and walnuts.

About a half hour after that you're washing dishes and suddenly feel dizzy, pass out, hit your head on the side of the kitchen cabinet knocking yourself out. You wake up with a lump on the side of your head and a sore hip, not knowing how long you've been out. Now you realize that due to CRS you've taken the blood pressure medication twice this morning.

Of course negativity sets in and you tell yourself that if you had died from that fall, someone would have found you eventually (you live alone).

Later in the morning when you've dusted yourself off and checked the mirror to see if you recognize yourself, you get dressed, throw the blood pressure pills out, and have a cup of ice-cream to chase away the gloom.

That doesn't help because the sugar rush gives you a vicious headache and your heart races like a freight train. So, you fish the blood pressure pills out of the garbage, have two glasses of water to try to flush out the ice-cream but that only makes the headache worse. Could this day get any worse? Oh, yeah, you get a notice that the rent for your government-subsidized apartment is going up $100 a month!.

Upside: While you're lying down trying to ease the headache and forget about the $100 rent increase, and Arthritis, UPS delivers a package to you from your daughter who lives in New Jersey now. Inside the package there's a Barbie Doll and a note that reads:

"Mommy, this is for you for all the times you didn't get to be a little girl."

Can anything so trivial as a lump on the head or a headache, a rent increase, or Arthritis mess with that? Ha Ha.

2.   It's not a particularly bad day starting out. You wake up as usual at 6 a.m., have a skimpy breakfast of toast, decaf green tea with honey, and half an apple.

It's three months into your retirement. You're learning to live on your social security and small pension, and you don't mind too much living alone.

You're planning to take a walk, but it starts pouring down rain just as you're getting dressed. Scratch that idea. You watch the morning talk shows, and *The Doctors*. By then you're beginning to feel kinda old, you know? No job, no phone calls, no letters from friends, or relatives who live far away. Watching *Shrek* again just makes you want to be in love too. You've been a widow for quite a few years now, and you figure if Shrek can find love, there's hope for you, despite your age of 75.

The pity party is in full swing by around 3:30 in the afternoon, and you're thinking, "Is there anybody out there as lonely as I am right now?"

When your cell phone rings you consider not even bothering to reach over from your dented spot on the sofa to grab it, but you do. In your most put-on happy voice you say "Hello." (Heaven forbid the person on the other end of the line should know that you're in the middle of one of your most successful pity parties.)

Your son is brief with his request: *"Can I make dinner reservations for three for tonight?"* (himself and two of his children)

There are two ways to respond to this request. 1) "I think you have the wrong number." 2) "What time, anything special?"

You choose 2).   A lifeline that would require all your attention for several hours; someone cares.

So after you halt the pity party, chase out all the negative thoughts and feelings, and put Arthritis on the back burner, you set to work planning a menu: Honey BBQ ribs, rice, canned green peas and kernel corn, French bread and butter, and raw vegetables with small cooked shrimp marinated in *Zesty Italian* salad dressing for appetizers. Ice-cream from the freezer for dessert.

Dinner turns out to be a pleasure, food spread all over the place and a big mess in the kitchen. Even clean-up isn't bad because when there are family dinners everyone helps with the clean-up.

By the time your dinner guests leave and you've put the kitchen in order, you're not even upset that Arthritis will try to follow you to bed, because you're fortified with the knowledge that you've just spent several hours with loved ones. You just take two *Anacin*® tablets to silence him.

And it's at least another week before the next pity party guests try to sneak back into your day.

3.   You wake up feeling blue one morning, and Arthritis is riding you as if you're a saddled pony. The only things on your body that don't hurt are your finger nails. It's too cold out to go for a walk. No one has called or written to you for over a week. The three friends you try to connect with are not answering their phone. You figure this is going to be a long, tough day.

You hobble to the medicine cabinet for your prescribed ass-kicker for Arthritis, get a cup of freshly-brewed coffee and a donut from your emergency freezer stash for days like this, and spend a few blessed hours with your friends around the world on *Blogit.com*. You get a dose of life lessons and humor while reading their blogs that brightens your day.

One of the blogs sends a powerful, profound message: "Don't ever lose your zest for life."

After your time on *Blogit* you watch The Jerry Springer show and feel fabulous about your life at 73. There was a woman on the show who was keeping her lover's artificial leg hostage because he already had a fiancée. And get this, that fiancée was also on the show dressed in a wedding dress, prepared for a wedding.

And there was another woman on the show dressed in a

wedding dress ready to marry her mama's boyfriend, but first she had a knock-down, drag out fight with the *boyfriend's* mother.

You laugh a lot, Arthritis takes a hike, and the blues vanish. Later that night you get another dose of *Blogit.com.*

4.   Arthritis takes a morning off, and when he shows up late afternoon, you kick his butt into oblivion with a cup of green tea, two *Tylenol® Extra Strength* pills, and *Shrek*

Although Arthritis is a monstrous burden to bear as you age, there are those mornings when you quietly accept the little twinges of pain when you first wake up, because it reminds you that you've been blessed with another day; *It beats the alternative any day.*

Laura from Connecticut says that she has accepted Arthritis as something that comes with aging. She says that if she ever wakes up one morning and doesn't have a single pain she'll just reach over for the phone and call the undertaker and reserve her place in line.

PART FOUR

Romance

1.   Dating Someone in Your Own Age Group

a) You will both probably move at the same pace, belch discreetly after a meal, and fall asleep in the middle of a movie or at the Opera

b) If a flatulent incident happens, there'll be no need for embarrassment or explanation, because you both have accepted them as bodily functions that may or may not occur at anytime

c) You can share reading glasses

d) Lovemaking is a *shared* pleasure because neither one of you has to try to show off

2.   Snuggling on the sofa with your partner on a snowy Saturday night with the sound of Kenny G's *Classics in the Key of G,* or Barry White's voice surrounding you. On the coffee table there's a tray that your partner put together, with your favorite sherry- - Harvey's Bristol Crème - -, cheese wedges, seedless green grapes, sliced apples, gourmet snack crackers, hot wings, and napkins with naughty pictures on them.
After the snack your partner squeezes you closer and whispers "I love you."

3.   A new lover. Someone who awakens all the first stirrings of passion from your first experience with love (and you both move at the same pace).

4.   Guilt-free afternoon naps snuggled up with your partner

5.   Spooning with your partner becomes special

6.   Sipping a glass of Harvey's Bristol Crème sherry in the evening with your partner's head in your lap

7.   Yoga, it's supposed to enhance your sex life

8.   Your partner has been working out at the gym (he's 74; you're about to knock 79 off your life's map). When he takes you out to dinner, the waitress and the coat-check girl flirt with him but you enjoy it because you know he's going home with you.

9.   You roll over in bed one morning and your partner is smiling at you. You realize they're thinking the same thing as you. You're both retired, you don't have to get up and go out into the cold, opinionated workforce. You can have brunch in bed, beginning with dessert, despite morning breath.

10.   Rainy Sundays with your partner, a pizza delivery, Columbo and Poirot DVD's, and a bottle of Hennessy

11.   Your volunteer assignment was especially difficult for you on a particular day because one of the patients at the rehab facility passed away. You drag yourself home dreading dinner preparations for your partner, who's working until 6:00.

You're in tears by the time you get home. As you enter the apartment, you get a whiff of an unbelievably wonderful aroma. Your partner meets you at the door with a glass of white wine, an embrace and a kiss that erases most of the past eight hours.

He's wearing a pair of skimpy shorts, a muscle shirt, and flip-flops that expose clean, pedicured feet. His all-grey hair is wet so you know he's just showered because his arms and legs are still glistening (he never towels himself dry because he says it dries up your skin, so he uses the damp washcloth).

"Dinner in 15 minutes," he says against your ear as he hugs you tighter, then kisses you again. "I left work early and I made your favorite, short ribs in that sauce you like, baked red potatoes and green peas."

After dinner he serves dessert in the bedroom with the smooth, soft sound of Clyde Terrell filling the room. Just before you pass out from exhaustion, you remind yourself that 75 is just a number! And this is not a dream.

12. You develop a crush on Dr. Oz when you hear him advise having sex at least twice a week to help reduce stress.
Bonus: When you tell your partner this, they agree!!

13. You've been a widow for three years, and at 77 possibilities for a second chance at love seem lost forever. But watching the news about the 85-year-old-Duchess of Alba's wedding to a much younger man gives you new hope.

And you're even more hopeful after watching an episode of *Divorce Court Before Your Vows.* A couple who had been together for 32 years wanted to get married, but needed Judge Toler's advice because they were having difficulties in their relationship and weren't sure if they should take that step.
After expressing their concerns and getting some much-needed, heartfelt advice from the Judge, she married them on the spot.

14. You're careful what you wish for. While in a heated argument with your partner you yell, "I wish you'd go somewhere and leave me alone."
The next day he has to go away on business for three weeks. You part without settling the argument.

Upside: After three days he calls to talk things over. You make up during the conversation and he says he can't stand being without you so you join him at the hotel for a week.

15. At 75 you're still working part-time as a waitress, and this Friday evening has been particularly gruesome because there was a committee meeting held in one of the special rooms at the restaurant.

There were 25 members attending, having a four-course meal. You and the other two waitresses received excellent tips, but that doesn't help your sore feet and back.

As you're leaving you find your partner waiting for you. He tells you he's booked a room at a hotel for a romantic week-end for the two of you. No phones, no cooking, no contact with anyone but the room service staff.

When you get to the room, you find he's packed a few of your personal things, there's a bottle of champagne and a little basket of gourmet snack foods, roses, and he says he's rented a naughty movie for the night.

Best of all, when you wake up the next morning you realize this was *not* a dream.

16.   Your partner had to break a dinner date because of problems at the office. It's the third time he's broken a date in the last four months. You control your anger and disappointment because he will be traveling on business for a week. After he's left you give in to the tears until you find a hastily-written poem from him in your underwear drawer:

> *No one else can take my stress or heartache away*
> *You make each and every day*
> *Count in so many special ways*
> *When things go wrong you make them right*
> *Without fuss or bother each day and night*
> *My heart belongs to you*

17.   After 35 years together your husband still likes to neck with you.

PART FIVE

A. Humorous CRS Episodes

1.   You go to the Mall to do some shopping. After shopping you're on the bus headed home and you reach in your purse for a tissue and discover the car keys, then remember that you drove to the Mall.

Upside: You remembered that in one of your shopping bags there's a bag of *Dove©* dark chocolate nuggets. So you hop off the bus at the next bus stop and take a leisurely walk back to the Mall (about a mile) while enjoying a few of your chocolates on the way. One of the chocolate wrappers has a message that says: '*Think positive*'. It makes you smile. Another wrapper says: '*Keep moving forward and don't look back*'.

2.   Opening the pantry to get rice and finding the milk you bought yesterday, but couldn't find this morning

3.   You're all ready to print information you found on the internet, so you plug in the printer and add paper and press a button. Nothing happens, so you unplug everything and plug them in again. Still nothing, no lights come on.

Just before you smash the printer to the floor, while complaining about how poorly-made all products are nowadays, a little voice tells you to try the *ON* button on the top of the printer.
Okay, you tell yourself, anybody can make that kind of mistake.

4.   You've put together your favorite recipe for baked chicken, seasoned with crushed fresh rosemary, crushed red peppers, and black pepper, with a red onion cut in pieces and stuffed inside, and under the skin on the wings, and thighs.

Your homemade dressing of olive oil, balsamic vinegar, Dijon mustard, pressed garlic, black pepper, and honey is set aside for basting.

You rub the chicken with a bit of olive oil, place it in an uncovered pan in the oven, and set the timer for half an hour for the first basting. When you go to check it when the timer goes off, you notice *you didn't remember to turn the oven on.*

Heck, you tell yourself, that's not as bad as putting on a pot of water to boil for tea and then going to the mall!

5.   Vanity is not a particularly strong part of your character and you rarely critique yourself in the mirror. You head out early one morning to go shopping. At the elevator you say good morning to a neighbor and she gives you a look that's a mixture of shock, humor, and pity. Okay, you tell yourself, maybe she's having a bad day already.

When the elevator gets to the ground floor another tenant that you see often stops you as you exit the elevator. "I think you forgot something," he says, pointing to your head.

You touch your hair and realize you forgot to comb your hair, and you must look like Don King's twin sister. Your hair is all gray in front and it's standing on end.

After you rush back to your apartment and comb your hair, you write a note on a big piece of paper that simply says: *Hair?,* and tape it to the front door along with the other notes that say: *shopping bags?; Shoes? Skirt?* (Since your skirt is usually the last thing you put on before leaving the house, you don't want a repeat of the time you left without putting it on. Luckily you were only standing outside the apartment door and happened to bend down to pick up the keys you dropped, and you were able to dart back inside the apartment to put on your skirt before anyone saw you.

And how about the time you got all the way to the corner bus stop before you realized you were still wearing your slippers.)

6.   One evening you come home late from a full day: a doctor visit in the morning; a four-hour volunteer assignment in the afternoon, and then grocery shopping.

You pop one of your prepared freezer dinners in the microwave for dinner. When the microwave signal sounds, you shut it off and take a quick shower.

Fifteen minutes later after your shower you get a call from a friend you haven't spoken to in weeks. While you're chatting with him you grab an apple and a health cookie to calm your rumbling stomach's hunger noises. After the phone call you're exhausted so you grab a glass of skim milk and go straight to bed.

The next morning when you open the microwave to heat water for instant coffee, you discover the dinner from the night before.

Okay, you tell yourself, at least you found it before it started to smell up the kitchen.

7.   Rushing to an early appointment one morning, you greet a neighbor in the elevator with a big smile. Your tongue touches a space in the front of your mouth and you realize you forgot to put in your partials.

The neighbor immediately takes out her full dentures and you both enjoy toothless grins and laughter before you rush back into your apartment for your partials.

8.   One morning you search for your partial dentures. You thought you'd left them to soak in the *Efferdent©* last night as usual. When you open the refrigerator an hour later, you find the dentures in there along with the glass and saucer you didn't feel like washing up after your Oreos and milk last night.

Okay, so what you tell yourself. At least this time you remembered to look for the partials *before* you went to the elevator. (*Karma* at work here. Remember how you used to laugh at your mom or grandmother when they'd be looking all around for their glasses, and all the while they were on the top of their head?)

9.   You're in a hurry one morning as you head out with a plastic

shopping bag with a few items you need to return to a department store, and a bag of garbage for the incinerator. The bags are almost the same size and weight.

On the first floor you drop what you believe is the garbage in the incinerator container, and head out to the bus stop. As you're stepping on the bus you notice the bag you're holding is actually the garbage.

Fortunately when you rush back to the incinerator room and claw through the garbage, the bag with your items is found in tact with just a little slime on the outside of the bag.

Okay you tell yourself, that's not so bad. Last week one night you took out chops for dinner and put them in the microwave to defrost. As you were about to set the controls on the microwave dial, the doorbell rings. On his way home your partner had ordered Chinese food for dinner so that you wouldn't have to cook.

The next morning when you open the microwave to heat the sausages for breakfast, the chops are thawed just enough to be prepared with a marinade for tonight's dinner. No real loss!

10.   You're getting ready one morning to head out to your volunteer assignment at a local nursing home. You lay out your outfit, which includes tights and a pair of tube socks to battle the 25-degree New York weather.

After you're dressed you sit down for a cup of tea and a slice of toast, then you spend a few minutes searching for the tube socks before you happen to glance down and notice you're wearing them.

Ok, that wasn't as bad as the time you got all the way to the nursing home before you noticed you still had your slippers on.

11.   You're doing a load of laundry one morning in the convenient laundry room on your floor in the senior hi-rise building. After you take the clothes out of the washing machine, you load them in the dryer and go back to your apartment and set the timer for 50 minutes. You get the clothes from the dryer when the time is up, and put them on the living room sofa to fold later, then you go to your bedroom and take a quick nap.

When you wake up from the nap you rush to the laundry room thinking you've forgotten your clothes, and find an empty dryer. Right away you think someone has *stolen* your laundry! You go back to your apartment and make yourself a fresh cup of coffee while tears are flowing and you're wondering why someone would do such an evil thing. "A bunch of nasty thieves," you wail, remembering that once before someone had stolen your laundry detergent. The tears flow and you boo-hoo for about ten minutes until you happen to go to the living room *and notice the clothes waiting on the sofa for you.*

You console yourself with a ten-minute spurt of laughter, and thank God that you didn't rush down to the security guard to report the *theft.*

12.   While going over what you believe to be your January, 2012 checking account statement you notice a charge you know nothing about. You call the number listed on the statement and ask the customer service representative to check it out for you.

After about 10 minutes of checking the account number and the transaction number, the mystery is solved; it was an on-line purchase from *2011*, a whole year ago.

After the call you send up a special prayer for the customer service rep who was so courteous and never once mentioned that the charge was made a year ago.

Okay, you tell yourself, it's the bank's fault for keeping all those files on-line, it's too confusing and anyone could make the same mistake.

B. <u>Managing CRS</u>

1. You keep a notebook in plain view at all times for notes to remind you to do something. You forget to do it anyway but when that little voice in your head speaks to you, you review your notes and catch up

2. During phone calls you jot down notes in a special notebook so that next time you talk to the same person you can just glance through the notes from the last conversation. (Your notebook is divided into sections with tabs that you have clearly marked)

3. Those little pill containers that separate your medications for each day really work!

4. When a doctor's appointment is scheduled, you immediately write it on a slip of paper and tape it to your closet door, AFTER you've added it to your personal calendar that's hanging on the wall *in* your closet

5. If you drive, you've learned *not* to place anything on top of the car so your hands are free to open the car door. You've seen the TV. commercial where the woman drives off while her coffee cup and papers fly off the top of the car. That only happened to you once though

6. You write the date on each slip of paper from your *choice jar* and recycle them so that you remember which activity you've done

7. To remember what name you've given your dolls and stuffed animals, you've slipped a name tag inside their clothes, or pinned it to them somewhere.

C. <u>Old-age Humor</u>

1.   Finding yourself talking to the cat as if it's a human being. When he responds to your chit-chat with various meows, you laugh it off and hope the neighbors didn't hear you

2.   Finding yourself practicing your frugal ex's habit of recycling toothpicks by soaking them in water (He also used to mail his bills without stamps until the post office started putting that note on envelopes that said a stamp was required.)

3.   Your 6-year-old grandson invents a game that he wants you to be the first one to play with him.

He says, "Granny I bet you can't last a whole day without saying the word *can't.*"

You lose in the first two seconds with your response: "I can't do that, how about half a day."

You have to join him when he starts to laugh at you.

<u>Warning</u>: If you get sucked into playing this game, don't bet money because you'll lose every time. You can practice alone, and for good brain activity add another word from the useless words and phrases list. It's fun and maddening at the same time.

PART SIX

A. Spirit Refreshers

1.   Phone calls out of the blue from family or friends

2.   Birthdays when people show up with food, cake, ice-cream, and gifts

3.   Charitable Donations - It feels good to share what you have, even if it's just a little bit of your little bit; and you'll soon notice that the more you give away the more you seem to have

4.   The smiles and warm hugs you get from an elderly friend who has no real family, when you visit them in the nursing home

5.   Fresh-brewed coffee and a chocolate-covered donut for breakfast

6.   Guilt-free indulgence in all things chocolate; it will never let you down

7.   Couch-potato days. Those intermittent days when the world seems to stop and you put a massive dent in the sofa with a Brenda Jackson novel, three DVD's: *Butterfield 8*, *Toy Story*, and *Somewhere in Time*, with an expensive bottle of wine, Chicken wings from the freezer, and whole wheat toast

8.   Having the family over for sundaes, with all the ingredients: three flavors of ice-cream, nuts, chocolate, whipped cream, cherries, strawberry syrup, chocolate fudge, etc.

9.   Learning that a dear friend who was very ill is getting better

10.   **Volunteering**

Helping others is a wonderful way to give back . It never fails to lift your spirits and boost your over-all good feeling when you know that you've helped someone. If you're blessed enough to be physically able to get around, imagine how someone who is house-bound feels not being able to get around. There are many ways to offer your services to other seniors:

a)   You can volunteer your services or particular talent at a nursing home, or senior center

b)   If you're a shopping aficionado, your volunteered services will be welcome to seniors who happen to be house-bound, or physically challenged

c)   If you like good conversation, you can share some of that with a house-bound senior who would enjoy discussing their interests

d)   The Meals On Wheels program can always use more help. For many seniors who receive deliveries from this program, it is the only time they have visitors.

11.   *Drop Dead Diva* on Sunday night

12   Rainy days with a Barbara Delinsky or a Lucinia Wright novel, a glass of cold milk and a gigantic chocolate chip cookie

13.   Lifetime movies, the kind that lets you imagine that you're the slim, beautiful heroine

14.   Music from artists from *your era* that you have on CD's

-Louis Armstrong
-Marvin Gaye
-Sonny & Cher
-Otis Redding
-The Monkeys

-Aretha Franklin
-The Beatles
-Gladys Knight and the Pips
-Ella Fitzgerald
-Frank Sinatra

-Dean Martin
-Sam Cooke
-Bing Crosby
-Tony Bennett
..... and so on.

15.   Gordon and Norma Yeager's story

In these troubled times of so much violence and economic horror stories, the story of this couple brings something so special to your heart and spirit.

They were married May 26, 1939, and after 72 years together, died within one hour of each other while still holding hands.

What a legacy they left behind for their children, grand children, great grand children, and great, great grand children.

16.   The episode of *Amazing Stories* entitled *Dorothy and Ben,* and *Boo!*

17.   Strangers who smile at you in passing

18.   An elderly friend who calls you an angel when you drop by to see her at the nursing home

19.   A friend who calls you up out of the blue and invites you to dinner with her and her adult son. You enjoy great food, easy-flowing conversation, and watching the camaraderie between your friend and her son. Even though your friend is more than 20 years your junior, they accept you as "good company".

20.   A week after you announce your pending retirement from your medical practice some of your patients show up at the office with gifts, food, and a cake to celebrate, and they bring along their children, that you delivered.

21.   Random acts of kindness

22.   *Nooners*. (Most spirit-refreshing when they're spontaneous).

23.   News of the rescue of a two-week-old from quake rubble of a Turkish apartment building.

B. Drug-free Stress Relievers

1.   All things chocolate

2.   Scrabble and Chinese Food with friends

3.   Brain teasers: Crossword puzzles; Sudoku, Jigsaw puzzles

4.   The Jerry Springer Show

5.   Late Night With Jimmy Fallon and his *Thank You Notes*

6.   Your favorite Psalm

7.   Paint-by-Number sets

8.   *Ellen;* you will not be able to resist the urge to dance

9.   Pbskids.org

10.   **Tears** --- How remarkable it is to be able to release the body's sorrow, mental anguish, and pain through these wonders. Whenever you feel the need to boo-hoo, you can let the tears flow freely, then watch the *Shrek* series to regain control. (Just be careful not to spend too much time in this boo-hoo shell because after a while the tears will begin to sap your energy.)

11.   **Feel-good books to keep in your nightstand drawer:**

--*Chicken Soup for the Soul - To Grandma, with Love* -- by Jack Canfield & Mark Victor Hansen

--*The Little Cold Book* --by Justin Spring (This will help calm you if you're nursing a cold, and the tips and recommendations will be a huge help fighting the cold.)

49

--*Celebrating Mothers* -- by Teri Wilhelms & Debbie Denton
(The title says it all, but the collection of tidbits is refreshing,
and enlightening.)

--*Cats - antics and attitudes* (If you've had a bad day, just
glance through this collection of cats of all kinds, with cute
captions and you'll laugh until you cry, then fall asleep happy.)

--*The Meaning of Life* -- by Bradley Trevor Greive
(This is an amazing collection of different species of life, with
comical and real explanations of their particular life)

12.   Mahalia Jackson music.

PART SEVEN

Learning new things

1.   Crater Lake in Oregon is the deepest lake in the U.S. - nearly 2000 feet deep

2.   Bread was invented by the Egyptians over 10,000 years ago

3.   Don't brush your teeth right after drinking red wine

4.   The Ostrich has the largest eyes of any land animal - - 2 inches across

5.   The only mammal that can't jump is an elephant

6.   The name of Patty Hearst's fiancé when she was kidnapped was Steven Weed

7.   Never eat raisins in the dark

8.   The Twinkie was invented in 1930

9.   Acronym for **Bible:**

    Basic
    Instruction
    Before
    Leaving
    Earth

10.   You know that it's okay to be a little flawed even though you're basically fabulous

11.   Maine is the only state that has one syllable in its name.

12.   There's been some controversy as to whether or not Wilma Flintstone's maiden name is Pebble or Slaghoople. Her old friend Greta Gravel remembers her as Wilma Pebble

13.   Betty Rubble's maiden name was Betty Jean McBricker

14.   By now you know that alcohol and sex do not work well together; someone invariably tires or falls asleep too quickly

15.   October 1st is the most common birthday in the U.S.

16.   The FDIC was created in 1933, and no depositor has ever lost a penny

17.   Only your own species will be able to hold a conversation with you, not your pet

18.   The YMCA (Young Men's Christian Association) was founded in London, England, on June 6, 1844

19.   The first YMCA for African Americans was founded in 1853 in Washington, D.C. by Anthony Brown, a freed slave

20.   As you grow older your ears continue to grow. All the more reason not to wear your hair too short

21.   Spirits bend and sometimes even break, but they are very seldom beyond repair

22.   <u>In 1918</u>

       -A first-class stamp only cost 3 cents
       -A loaf of bread cost 10 cents
       -A gallon of milk cost 55 cents
       -A dozen eggs cost 37 cents
       -The average yearly income was $1,115 (In 1960 your annual

income was a whopping $3,200.)

23.   Chocolate and a little meditation will help you get through almost anything

24.   At age 79, if you have the slightest bit of a problem with your equilibrium, you don't do stupid shit like trying to put on your underwear, a skirt or half slip by stepping into it while standing. You now know that the best way to put on these items of clothing is to *sit down* and pull them up over your ankles, *then* stand up and pull them the rest of the way up.

25.   You know now not to watch *Days of Our Lives* every day if you're not getting any on a regular basis

26.   The ballpoint pen was invented by Laszio Biro in 1935

27.   Ruth Handler invented the Barbie Doll in 1959

28.   The band-aid was invented by Earle Dickson in 1921

29.   The Oreo Cookie was invented by Nabisco in 1912

30.   The lemon squeezer was invented by John Thomas White

31.   The pop-up toaster was invented by Charles P Strite in 1919

32.   Velcro was invented by Georges de Mestral in 1941

33.   Your partner *does so* know when you're faking it

34.   Elephants give themselves dust baths to help protect them from the sun

35.   Oliver Lewis won the first Kentucky Derby in May, 1875

36.   Put your dentures in *as soon as you get out of bed*, that way you won't forget them

37.   Young kangaroos are called joeys.

PART EIGHT

General Upsides

1.   Computers and the Internet

If you happen to have a computer and are willing to open yourself up to new experiences (not too much, but just enough to be able to enjoy the entertainment), you can spend hours on the internet corresponding with friends around the world at different sites like *Facebook, Blogit.com,* and others

And if you're computer-savvy, you can have hours of fun with sites like *Virtual World,* and *You tube.*

2.   Occasional Solitude

a)   If you happen to be single and living alone, there are those times when blessed solitude hugs you like a favorite sweater: No husband to ask where his supper is, or where you put his socks; no children to take to school; no grandchildren to baby sit; nothing at all to prevent you from lounging on the sofa watching TV or movies all day, with chips and ginger-ale; or spending the day with a good book.

And later in the evening you grab remnants from the fridge or freezer, have a glass of wine, surf the net for hours, then fall into bed exhausted and you fall asleep in a blessed old-age cloud of joy.

This kind of thing happens now and then, mostly <u>THEN</u> Ha Ha. Because when you wake up the next day after all that solitude, you go outside and start talking to strangers because you realize the people on the TV. or in the movies or books can't have a conversation with you. And all your cat's meows are starting to sound alike.

So you call up a friend who's also retired and you both go to the casino and blow some of your social security or pension checks on the slot machines.

b)   You can still have solitude whenever you damn well please, even if your partner "...doesn't understand". And if at anytime the solitude begins to get you down, there's always your *choice jar*.

3.   The TV/DVD Remote Control

How many times have you grabbed the TV remote control device so you wouldn't have to listen to the same commercial that's already interrupted your one-hour program 3 times in the first half-hour?

You can thank A. Robert Adler for inventing the first wireless TV. Remote control device in 1956. Now you can just switch the channel whenever that annoying little bear decides to wipe his butt and discuss the strength of toilet tissue during your favorite program.

After you switch channels, if you're experiencing CRS you won't remember which program you were watching anyway, so don't worry.

4.   Breaking the rules without a care in the world because you know you've *paid your dues*

5.   Knowing that treating yourself is never wrong

6.   Musical Sounds

-The tinkly laugh of a baby

-The snickering laugh of a kid when you tell them a corny joke

-That special *Meow, or Woof* sound your pet makes when they want to tell you they love you

-The sound of the voice of one of your grown children on the phone

-"I love you, Granny," from a five-year-old grandson

-Your partner's "Ummm." in your ear when they hug you

-The sound of the coffee perculator in the morning

-The soft sound of raindrops against your window on a spring night

-The ring of the phone interrupting a pity party when it's *not* a wrong number.

7.   Kindle/Nook Reading devices

Electronic reading devices are one of man's most treasured inventions besides the internet (for some of us). You can carry your own personal library around with you at all times, read where and when you want to, even share your library with others who happen to have the same device as yours, and vice-versa.

Recently Kindle announced they're working with public libraries for a lending program for the device.

And if you don't prefer the portable device, you can download the programs for these devices for free, and store your library on your computer.

8.   Finding new scrabble words

9.   Digital Cameras - - They're small enough to fit right in your purse or pocket, so that you can review precious pictures of your family or friends anytime you want while on the go

10.   At this age you can tell *Fear* to kiss your butt

11.   Columbo DVD's

12.   Agatha Christie mysteries

13.   Your secret, hopeless crush on Leland Stottlemeyer from the *Monk* TV. show (played so convincingly by Ted Levine)

14.   Netflix

You can stream movies and episodes of your favorite TV. shows - - old and new - - to your TV., or computer. You get to see lots of the old TV. shows and black and white classic movies, the kind where romance is *implied* and you get to use your imagination for the rest, according to your own personal idea of romance.

Rose says *An Affair to Remember* is the most romantic movie she's ever seen.

15.   Blockbuster on Demand

With this service, you can order a movie on-demand, with some prices as low as $1.99 per movie

16.   Calling the Customer Service department of a particular company and actually hearing a *human* voice on the other end of the line

17.   Lifelock

 Even before this age you were susceptible to identity theft

18.   Lifeline

If you've ever fallen and had trouble getting up, you've long since stopped snickering at the commercial where the woman is lying on the floor saying, "I've fallen and I can't get up."

19.   Cell Phones - What on earth did we ever do before them?

BUT   We also send up a daily prayer that a Federal law will be passed to outlaw cell phone use on public transportation

20.   The Wendy Williams Show -   It's not gossip, it's a healthy interest in human behavior

21.   Peapod Grocery Delivery

22.   A *Kitchen Sink Pizza* delivered to your door from *Fellini Pizzeria* (In Providence, RI.) It's a meal in a box: "*Penne pasta, spinach, feta cheese, scallions, roasted red peppers, topped with pepperoni and parmesan peppercorn sauce.* " all baked on a thin crust

23.   Chicken wings, a chef salad, and garlic bread, delivered to your door from *Sicilia's Pizzeria - - Home of the Famous stuffed Pizza.* (In Providence, RI)

24.   Making your own rules

25.   <u>**Mother Nature**</u>

She doesn't have to explain herself. Her existence is just one of those things in life you can never hope to explain, or understand. Sort of like the *Incredible Hulk* who always manages to keep his pants on while all his other clothes get ripped away when he changes from David Banner to the *Hulk.*

You can either take Mother Nature or leave her; if you decide to leave her, just go quietly. But if you decide to stick around, her weather shenanigans notwithstanding, she never lets you down or fails to dazzle you with some of her magic.

After she's sprinkled rain to wash away all the dog poop that uncaring, disgusting pet owners leave on the streets, she puts on a show for you when you're out for a walk:

--Every tree is dressed differently in their own unique style for spring

--Besides your partner's smile, try to think of something with more natural, fleeting beauty than a multi-colored fall leaf that lands near your feet

--A rainbow with its vibrant colors, red, orange, yellow, green, blue, indigo, and violet.

--The intoxicating smell of freshly-cut grass

--The first flowers' bloom

--150-year-old trees that defy every scientific study

--The musical sound of the cricket's mating calls

--Catching snowflakes on your tongue

       Even in the confines of your home, she dazzles you with her magic:

--The sound of the first bird's song of spring waking you up in the morning

--A pigeon's soft coo when it lands on your window sill

26.   Having the time to read Nathaniel Hawthorne, August Wilson, and William Shakespeare

27.   Judge Mathis; Judge Joe Brown; Judge Judy; Judge Pirro; Judge Toler

28.   Young men who offer you their seats on a crowded bus

29.   Bus drivers who request that younger people give up the seat that's intended for the elderly or handicapped

30.   People who sit beside you at the bus stop and ask if the smoke will bother you *before* they light up

31.   Weight Watchers on-line

32.   Being able to *clip* out the bad memories from your past and only keeping the good ones to go over every once in a while

33.   Eyebrow threading by a professional (no more pinched skin when you try to pluck them yourself)

34.   One Saturday you pick *Folderol* from your choice jar, and you explore new places in your city. You visit stores in the Malls and window-shop. It's a warm day so you stroll around the city and sit in the park reading.

        When you return home you realize you've seen more male underwear in four hours than you've probably seen of your husband's underwear during the first year of your marriage. This is because most of the young men you saw today wore their pants *drooping* half-way down their butts. And this makes them walk weird, as if they're carrying a load in their pants.

        You've heard that in one state this is a misdemeanor. After discussing it with a neighbor, you both begin writing letters to your Alderman, your City Councilman, the Mayor, and Governor, asking for the passing of a law to make this practice a misdemeanor for public indecency in your state.

35.   Conversation

        In this electronic age of Texting, E-mail, Facebook, and Twitter, the actual sound of a human voice can seem like a miracle.

        Even trying to get *customer service* from companies through speaking to a human being can be frustrating. Most of the time you have to listen to the computerized instructions to *"press one for..."* and so on, and by the time you get to speak to a human being you hang up the phone because CRS has taken over and you've forgotten why the hell you called in the first damn place.

--We Text our loved ones and friends and add smiley faces with hearts, and x's and o's, more often than we telephone

--We E-mail with important information and upcoming events, and send pictures

--We go back and forth with our friends on Facebook

--We twitter with news, and *follow* friends and celebrities

Thanks to these forms of communication face-to-face *conversation* is becoming something as rare as a drive-in movie place. No wonder you behave as if you've won a million-dollar lottery when you actually hear the voice of a loved one on the other end of the telephone.

Upside: To maintain connection with your own species (You've been having conversations with the cat a lot lately) you make a list of everyone you're acquainted with in any way, and you call someone on the list often, especially when the pity party guests are clamoring at your door to get in. And if you forget where you left the list last, just call the first person whose name pops into your head.

36.   Family and friends who treat you like a person instead of a troublesome old lady

37.   Living your dream whatever it may be, despite the sometimes negative comments from others

38.   **Economy and Frugality**

You've learned several tricks to lessen the strain on your budget by:

--Keeping a container of those left-over *spoonfuls* of vegetables in the freezer for making soup

--Unplugging regular appliances and electronics when they're not in use:
          -The VCR
          -The microwave

-The Toaster, or Toaster oven
-The coffee maker
-The AC
-The TV.

--Shredded documents/personal papers make excellent packing material

--When you can't pump any more lotion or shampoo out of a container, you cut it in half and find you have enough to transfer to a smaller container

--Melting those little pieces of soap together to make one full colorful bar

--Using the funny papers to wrap gifts

39.   When you get tired of watching the cast of *Days Of Our Lives* having sex you:

--Call a friend and go out to the movies and dinner

--Read a book from your Kindle library, or one from your personal hard-copy library

--Visit a friend who's in a nursing home, and take them a little goodie

--Volunteer to help out a neighbor who has been ill, or who has had a family emergency

--Cook a fantastic meal and invite some family or friends over

40.   <u>Feel-good movies</u>

-Toy Story
-Shrek
-Finding Nemo

-An Affair to Remember
-The Kid

-Last Holiday
-Cinderella (No matter which version you watch)
-Why Did I Get Married
-The Princess and the Frog
-Ice Age

-Alvin and the Chipmunks

41.   **Feel-good TV. shows** (from your era) --They can be found
on Me TV. (Memorable Entertainment TV.); Nick at Nite, and other
cable channels, or on DVD

-Family Affair
-The Jeffersons
-The Mary Tyler Moore Show
-The Dick Van Dyke Show
- I Love Lucy

-The Beverly Hillbillies
-Good Times
-Petticoat Junction
-All in the Family
-The Golden Girls

-My Three Sons
-Love American Style
-The Odd Couple
-Green Acres
-Third Rock from the Sun

-Are You Being Served
-Fresh Prince of Bel-Air

42.   **Perspicacity:** Cultivate it, it'll help you cope with life

43.   <u>**Persnickety**</u>: You've earned the right, but be kind.

MOMMY-ISMS
(MOM'S UNFORGETTABLE PEARLS OF WISDOM)

1.   If   ifs and ands were pots and pans, they'd make a whole kitchen

2.   You don't trouble trouble, if trouble don't trouble you

3.   There's sunshine in every smile, even yours, so flaunt it

4.   Two wrongs don't make a right

5.   If you decide to seek revenge, dig two graves

6.   *Learn to forgive!* While you're wasting your life holding a grudge, that person has all but forgotten about you

7.   Forgiveness is the best revenge

8.   Learn to love the person in the mirror, with all their shortcomings

9.   When you want to critique someone, start with the person in the mirror

10.   Eat less and move more if you want to lose weight

11.   Riding on a high horse all the time can become unbearably lonely, so learn to walk on solid ground beside your fellow man

12.   Better to have loved and lost than never to have loved at all is a crock of bullshit

13.   You *can* love two partners at one time so long as one of them is the person in the mirror

14.   Smiles are free whether given or received, and they benefit your soul and your physical body

15.   Nothing compares to Mother Nature's nectar to quench your thirst

16.   Friends come and go but family is forever

17.   The dog that brings the bone of gossip will carry one back

18.   *Things* can be replaced when they're broken, but not people

19.   Like music, smiles are a universal language

20.   Don't tempt Ms. Fate, mind your business and your P 's and Q's.

21.   No one buys the cow if they can get the milk for free

22.   Once you leave don't go back because you'll find the same thing you left there, only it'll be worse

23.   *Think* before you speak because words once spoken in anger hurt forever

24.   Loneliness is a dirty word, so defy it by taking advantage of every free moment to:

     -Call a friend or relative
     -Read an uplifting book
     -Watch an uplifting movie, preferably *Shrek, Finding Nemo, Cinderella, Shark Tale, Alvin and the Chipmunks,* etc.

25.   Most of the time you need to keep your mouth shut and your eyes and ears open

26.   If you can't be content alone in your own company, it might be difficult for others to enjoy your company

27.   Trying to refine, re-shape, improve, re-invent or change your chosen partner is like trying to un-ring a bell

28.   By sharing your happiness you increase it many times over

29.   When you're feeling lonely or neglected, send someone you love this message: "I'm free today, so send me all your worries, burdens, and anxieties and I'll carry them for you all day."

30.   After the chase when your partner has finally caught you, work hard to keep the intrigue alive

31.   If you lie down with dogs you get up with fleas; gender doesn't matter, nor does it matter if the dogs walk on four legs or two

32.   If something's not broke, don't fix it

33.   If you don't like the person in your mirror, don't expect others to either

34.   Make kindness the hallmark of your personality.

FINALLY

1.   You're a year into your retirement, and have adjusted well to the change. You're using your *choice jar,* getting together with other retired friends, calling people from your list, volunteering, and enjoying your approach to old age.

When the phone rings now sometimes you tsk-tsk and wonder if you have time for a chat. Once or twice you actually have to beg a rain-check for a social invitation.

2.   You don't worry about things that are beyond your ability to control, like:

--Who your children or grand children fall in love with and choose as a mate

--The national debt

--Rising gas prices

--The man you saw coming out of your neighbor's apartment at six o'clock this morning (her husband is away on business)

3.   You live your life believing *everything* is a miracle

4.   You've set down your bag of bricks of guilt, envy, longing, vengeful thoughts for past slights or wrongs, etc., etc.

5.   You embrace those periods of solitude because the choice is yours; you know that you can make contact with *someone* from your list when you're ready, and you remain open to contact from others

6.   By now you're secure in the belief that *if/when* negatives do enter your life you will be fortified with all your upsides and positives to life after 70

7.   It's been 10 years since you emerged from the alcoholic haze you spent most of your life in, and your family still lets you share in their lives; *God was in the plan*

8.   By now you've learned not to waste time going back and wishing this or that had been different. *Would-da, Should-da, Could-da* are very rarely included in your vocabulary

9.   You know that this is your life now, and you intend to enjoy it by living it to the fullest. You intend to remind yourself often to live in the moment. And you've vowed to try to make happiness your choice, every day

10.   You've found out that the more you celebrate your life after 70, the more things you find to celebrate

11.   More and more you find yourself forgetting the rules and playing by your heart

12.   You notice that sharing your happiness with others never lessens it; it comes back two-fold every time you share it

13.   You find yourself enjoying the simple pleasures in life more and more each day

14.   You administer chocolate therapy for the slightest annoyance

15.   There's no space in your heart for anger, animosity, or thoughts of revenge for wrongs done to you, so you do all things with love

16.   By now you know that *every* problem has a solution; it just takes a little work to find it

17.   You often try to remember to discard a few useless, and discouraging words and phrases from your vocabulary that hinder or block your enjoyment of your everyday life:

--Can't (the worst offender)
--Couldn't
--Could've
--Hate (very toxic and contagious)
--If (sometimes)
--Maybe
--Never
--Should've
--Used to
--Was (sometimes)
--Would've

18.   You've adopted a *Will Rogers* philosophy; if you meet someone whose lifestyle or perceptions you disagree with, you don't waste precious time or brain activity criticizing them; you accept that they are different; and maybe you can learn something from them

19.   By now you've learned to live in the moment; you know there's no possible way to fix or undo past mistakes, or to predict the future

20.   You frequently take a look at your life and count your blessings and keep your complaints and grumblings about not having this or that to a bare minimum. If you don't like something about your life you change it if you can, and often gain a new appreciation for your life

21.   You live from your heart because by now you know it'll never steer you wrong.

22.   CRS has become just another annoyance, like the dust on the chandelier that you can never seem to get off.

23.   You still pray for a Mustang Ranch for women.

THE BEST UPSIDES/POSITIVES TO LIFE AFTER 70

When one of your little grown-up darlings:

a.   Calls because they *need* you for whatever the reason

b.   When they come by with Chinese food, a birthday cake, and gifts

c.   When they send you a Barbie Doll with a love note

d,   When they send you an uplifting text message when you're feeling low

e.   When they invite you out to dinner

f.   When they invite you to their house for a visit

Except for this:

You woke up this morning!!! (This is our favorite)

You get to make the day your own special miracle. You get to choose without asking anyone else's opinion:

a) Oh, woe is me. Another day.

b) Yippee! Another day!!!

****

Medicine For Your Taste Buds©

(From Rose and some of her friends)

1. <u>Trail mixes</u>

a. Serving-size portions of:

> --Cheerios
> --raisins
> --walnuts, chopped
> --mini marshmallows

b. Serving-size portions of:

> --*Whole Grain Total* cereal
> --Raisins
> --Chopped walnuts (or almonds)
> --*Cheerios*
> --*Trix* cereal

2. <u>Dark Chocolate Energy Bars</u>

> --Melt *Dove ®* chocolate in the microwave
> --Add chopped almonds (or walnuts)
> --Add Bran cereal

--Cool, then cut into blocks; keep refrigerated

3. <u>Oven-fried chicken</u>

-Preheat oven @ 350°

-Remove skin from chicken pieces

73

-Brush pieces evenly with olive oil
-Roll in seasoned cornflakes crumbs*
-Bake on lightly-greased cookie sheet at 350° for one hour

*Cornflakes crumbs:

--Crush about three cups of cornflakes
--Season with black pepper, crushed red pepper, fresh basil and thyme.

NOTE: Discard cornflakes crumbs after use.

4.   **Liver Slivers**

--3 slices frozen beef liver, thinly sliced into long slivers
--1 small red onion, thinly sliced
--3 tablespoons olive oil
--2 tablespoons low sodium soy sauce
--1 / 2 teaspoon raw sugar
--1 pat butter
--Black pepper, paprika, to taste

--Heat skillet, add oil, liver and onion
--Cook over high flame for about three minutes, just long enough for the liver to turn brown

--Remove skillet from burner, add soy sauce, raw sugar, butter, black pepper, and paprika

--Let stand for about two minutes

--Serve over brown rice
--Use leftovers cold over salads, or sprinkle in hot soup

5.   **Pickled Mushrooms**

--Rinse mushrooms thoroughly and gently remove stems (optional)
--Place mushroom caps in enough green tea to cover them, add a dash of raw sugar
--Bring to a rapid boil, for about two minutes
--Remove mushrooms from water and set aside to cool

--Place cooled mushrooms in a dish of *Robust Italian Salad Dressing*
--Marinate in refrigerator for 3 to 4 hours
--Pierce mushrooms with fork often so that the dressing goes through

6.   **Whole Grain Raisin Muffins**

--Preheat oven @ 400°

--1 cup unsifted *King Arthur* © whole wheat flour
--1-1/2 cups *Whole Grain Total* © cereal
--1 Tsp. baking powder
--1 /2 Tsp. nutmeg
--1/3 cup brownulated sugar
--2/3 cups *Dole* sun dried raisins

--1 egg
--1/4 cup vegetable oil (or extra light olive oil)
--1-1/4 cup skim milk

In small bowl:

--Mix together: flour, cereal, baking powder, nutmeg,

sugar, and raisins

In large bowl:

--Beat egg well
--Add oil, and skim milk - mix well

--Stir in dry ingredients just until well moistened

--Let mixture sit for about 4 to 5 minutes
--Lightly grease muffin wells (or use muffin cups); fill evenly

--Bake for approximately 20 to 25 minutes

--Yield: 12 muffins

NOTE: The dry ingredients in this recipe can be mixed together and kept in the refrigerator in a sealed container for up to three weeks, and will still be fresh, making it easy to have fresh muffins for breakfast in a flash.

****